Muhammad Fidel Ganis Siregar

The Role of Testosterone In Menopause

Muhammad Fidel Ganis Siregar

The Role of Testosterone In Menopause

General Management And Sexual Dysfunction Treatment

LAP LAMBERT Academic Publishing

Impressum / Imprint
Bibliografische Information der Deutschen Nationalbibliothek: Die Deutsche Nationalbibliothek verzeichnet diese Publikation in der Deutschen Nationalbibliografie; detaillierte bibliografische Daten sind im Internet über http://dnb.d-nb.de abrufbar.
Alle in diesem Buch genannten Marken und Produktnamen unterliegen warenzeichen-, marken- oder patentrechtlichem Schutz bzw. sind Warenzeichen oder eingetragene Warenzeichen der jeweiligen Inhaber. Die Wiedergabe von Marken, Produktnamen, Gebrauchsnamen, Handelsnamen, Warenbezeichnungen u.s.w. in diesem Werk berechtigt auch ohne besondere Kennzeichnung nicht zu der Annahme, dass solche Namen im Sinne der Warenzeichen- und Markenschutzgesetzgebung als frei zu betrachten wären und daher von jedermann benutzt werden dürften.

Bibliographic information published by the Deutsche Nationalbibliothek: The Deutsche Nationalbibliothek lists this publication in the Deutsche Nationalbibliografie; detailed bibliographic data are available in the Internet at http://dnb.d-nb.de.
Any brand names and product names mentioned in this book are subject to trademark, brand or patent protection and are trademarks or registered trademarks of their respective holders. The use of brand names, product names, common names, trade names, product descriptions etc. even without a particular marking in this work is in no way to be construed to mean that such names may be regarded as unrestricted in respect of trademark and brand protection legislation and could thus be used by anyone.

Coverbild / Cover image: www.ingimage.com

Verlag / Publisher:
LAP LAMBERT Academic Publishing
ist ein Imprint der / is a trademark of
OmniScriptum GmbH & Co. KG
Bahnhofstraße 28, 66111 Saarbrücken, Deutschland / Germany
Email: info@lap-publishing.com

Herstellung: siehe letzte Seite /
Printed at: see last page
ISBN: 978-3-659-82953-6

Copyright © 2016 OmniScriptum GmbH & Co. KG
Alle Rechte vorbehalten. / All rights reserved. Saarbrücken 2016

DEDICATION

I dedicate this book to my Mama and Papa, Selly, Ernesto, and Alessandro

ACKNOWLEDGEMENT

Special thanks to: Marah Ganti Siregar MD, Senior Lecturer in Pathology Anatomy, as a father and teacher as well as a pioneer founder of Faculty of Medicine Universitas Sumatera Utara, who guided me during the writer's life from childhood to the present. Professor Delfi Lutan MD MSc as a teacher, researcher, Consultant in Reproductive Endocrinology and Fertility Medicine, and currently as the head of the department of obstetrics & gynecology Faculty of Medicine Universitas Sumatera Utara, who has done a lot to make the author to become a gynaecologist, consultant in Reproductive Endocrinology and Fertility medicine, and until getting a Doctoral Degree in Medicine, and also taught the author to become a leader. Also to Yufi Permana Marsal, MD, Lydia Irtifany Lubis, MD, Iman Syahputra MD, Cherry Kumalasari, MD who have helped to finish up this writings.

ABSTRACT

Menopause is a normal, natural phase which occurs in all women. During the transition period from reproductive age to menopausal age, women experience a lot of physical changes. Even though many women go through menopause without any symptoms, or less disturbance in their daily lives, some experience major symptoms till the extend that it disrupts their quality of their lives. The major symptoms are changes in menstrual cycles, hot flushes, disturbed sleep, night sweats, dry vagina and reduction in sexual desire. The age of menopause is approximately from 45 years old till 55 years old. A few downside of menopause are reduction in libido, tiredness, reduction in sexual activity, which is caused by reduced testosterone level which starts to reduce since the woman is 20 years old. Due to the aging process which is followed by the reduction in steroid sex hormones in the circulation (estrogen, progesterone, testosterone), many researches has a hypothesis that the reduction in hormones help the degeneration and pathology related to the age. When the women reaches the age 45 years old, the testosterone level reduces 50%. A few researches concludes that the effectivity of testosterone treatment, uses the mood parameter, vitality and positive changes was reported in post menopausal women who uses testosterone.

Key word : Menopause, Sexual Dysfunction, Testosterone.

TABLE OF CONTENTS

DEDICATION i

ACKNOWLEDGEMENT ii

ABSTRACT iii

TABLE OF CONTENTS v

CHAPTER I INTRODUCTION 1

CHAPTER 2 MENOPAUSE 3
    2.1 Definition 3
    2.2 Physiology of Menopause 3
    2.3 Role of Activin and Inhibin in Molecular Menopause 7
    2.4 Clinical Manifestation of Menopause 17
    2.5 Osteoporosis in Menopausal Women 18
    2.6 Menopause Rating Scale (MRS) 25

CHAPTER 3 GENERAL MANAGEMENT OF MENOPAUSAL
WOMEN AND ROLE OF TESTOSTERONE IN MENOPAUSE 28
    3.1 General Management Of Menopausal Women 28
    3.2 Role Of Testosterone In Menopause 31
    3.3 Use of Testosterone in Menopausal Hormone Therapy 37

CHAPTER 4 CONCLUSION 47

AUTHOR 49

REFERENCES 50

CHAPTER 1
INTRODUCTION

Menopause is a normal and natural phase that happens to women. The ovary progessively fail to produce estrogen dan other hormones. Menopause indicates the permanent ending of the fertile state. During the transition period from reproductive age to menopausal age, women undergo many physical changes. Most of the changes are natural consequences due to both aging and menopause itself. Even though all woman undergo menopause, each has their own unique way.[1]

Most women experience menopause without any symptoms, and only slight disturbance in daily life. However, there are many woman that has severe symptoms which greatly influences their daily lives. There are many physical changes during menopause, caused by both menopause and aging. Some of them are, changes in menstrual cycle, hot flushes, disturbance is sleep, nocturnal sweating, dry vagina dan reduction in sexual function.[1]

Women normally undergo menopause between the age 45 till the age 55. Some of the major downside of menopause manifestation are reduced libido, tiredness, reduced sexual activity which is caused by the reduction of testosterone since the age 20 years old.[2,3]

Sex steroid hormone plays a very important role in upholding both reproductive and non reproductive function. Due to the aging process followed by the reduction of sex steroid hormone, many researches has a hypothesis that the reduction of these hormones helps the degeneration and pathology related to the age. By the age of 45 years old, the testoterone reduces around 50%.[3,4,5]

The role of testosterone androgen is already understood : it is importance toward the sexual arousal, vibration and receiving sexual stimulant.[2,5]

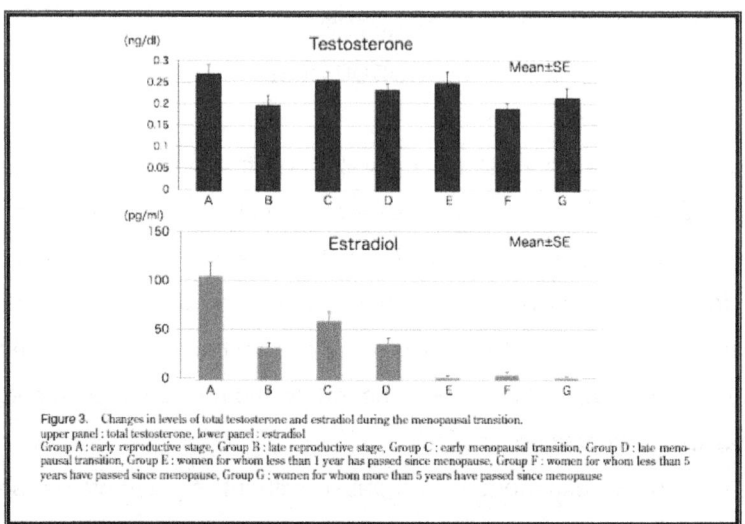

Figure 1. Chart of Changes in Level of Total Testosterone and Estradiol during The Menopausal Transition Period[6]

A few researches concludes that the efectivity of testosterone treatment using the mood parameter, vitality dan positive changes was reported in post menopausal women who uses testosterone.[3]

CHAPTER 2

MENOPAUSE

2.1. Definition

According to WHO, menopause is the cessation of the menstruation cycle forever for women who had period monthly before, caused by the increasing numbers of follicles undergoing atresia until there is no more follicle left, and for the last 12 months do experience amenorrhea that was not caused by pathological causes. Nowadays, Indonesian women experience menopause at approximately age 50. Nevertheless, some experience it in the early or late age. Age timing of menopause is influenced by heredity, general health status, an life style.[7-10]

2.2. Physiology of Menopause

The cause of the cessation of menstruation is due to the ovaries that no longer produce and release estrogen and progesterone hormones. *Webster's Ninth New Collegiate Dictionary* defines menopause as a period of the cessation of menstruation which is naturally occurred between the ages of 45 and 50. Menopause is the final bleeding from the uterus which is still influenced by hormones from the brain and the ovum.[7]

Menopause occurs because the production of the ovum runs at all and usually occurs between the ages of 45 and 50. The diagnosis is made after there was amenorrhea (no menstruation) at least for 1 year. *Shimp & Smith* defines menopause as the end of menstrual period, but a woman isn't considered in a postmenopause state until she has amenorrhea at least for the last 1 year. This cessation could be preceded by a longer period cycle with less bleeding. Usually, the lowest limit of the age of menopause is 44 years. Surgery or radiation may cause menopause with more complaints compared to the natural one.[7]

The last phase after the reproductive period expired is called climacterium, a transitional period a woman passed from the reproductive to the non-productive period. This period is lasting between 5 and 10 years or between 5 years before the menopause and 5 years after that. The climacterium period consists of three phases, those are premenopause, perimenopause, and postmenopause. The premenopause is the period before the perimenopause occurs. This period occurs since the reproductive function is getting decreased until the complaints or the menopause symptoms appear. The perimenopause is the period when the complaints peak. It occurs about 1-2 years before and 1-2 years after the menopause. The postmenopause is the period after the perimenopause until the senile period. In general, the climacterium phase is called as menopause.[7]

The production of female hormones (estrogen) is getting decreased so that the menstruation becomes irregular and eventually stops. After age of 40, a woman enters climacterium phase, which is derived from the word *climacter* that means transitional years. Climacterium or steady age, occurs since premenopausal period (approximately at age of 40) when the function of the ovaries was gradually decreased and ends approximately at 55 years. At age about 49 years, menopause (no menses) occurs.[7,8]

Menopause is a phase of a woman's normal life. In the menopausal period, a woman's reproductive capacity stops. The ovaries no longer function, the production of steroid hormones and peptides gradually disappears, and there is a number of physiological changes. Mostly are caused by the cessation of the ovarian function and the rests are caused by aging process. Many women experience symptoms and complaints as the results from the changes mentioned before. Those symptoms and complaints normally disappear gradually. Even though those can't lead to death, those provoke such an uncomfortable feeling and sometimes cause some interferes in daily works.[7]

Since being born, a female baby has about 770.000 undeveloped ova. In the puberty phase, at age of 8-12 years, it begin showing the light activity of the reproductive endocrine function. At the age of 12-13, generally a woman will get *menarche* (the first menses), known as puberty. At that time, the female reproductive organs are getting start to function optimally. The ovaries begin releasing ovum that are ready to be fertilized, called the reproductive phase or fertile period which is lasting until about 45 years of age. When the ova get fertilized at the fertile period, the pregnancy will occur.[7]

Menopause usually occurs at the age of late 40s or early 50s. According to WHO, menopause is the permanent cessation of menstruation caused by loss of ovarian follicular activity in which estrogen is secreted by ovarian primodial follicles. Although the ovaries of *eumenorrheic* contains an average of 1.000 follicles, during the transitional period (the perimenopause), the numbers of these follicles will be reduced by about 10-fold, and almost no follicles were found in the postmenopausal ovaries. The mechanisms of the follicle reduction and menopause are unknown.[7]

Table 1. The Chart of The Female Reproductive Stage[11]

Stage	-5	-4	-3b	-3a	-2	-1	+1a	+1b	+1c	+2
Terminology	REPRODUCTIVE				MENOPAUSAL TRANSITION		POSTMENOPAUSE			
	Early	Peak	Late		Early	Late	Early			Late
						Perimenopause				
Duration	variable				variable	1-3 years	2 years (1+1)		3-6 years	Remaining lifespan
PRINCIPAL CRITERIA										
Menstrual Cycle	Variable to regular	Regular	Regular	Subtle changes in Flow Length	Variable Length Persistent ≥7-day difference in length of consecutive cycles	Interval of amenorrhea of ≥60 days				
SUPPORTIVE CRITERIA										
Endocrine FSH AMH Inhibin B			Low Low	Variable Low Low	↑Variable Low Low	↑>25 IU/L** Low Low	↑Variable Low Low	Stabilizes Very Low Very Low		
Antral Follicle Count			Low	Low	Low	Low	Very Low	Very Low		
DESCRIPTIVE CHARACTERISTICS										
Symptoms						Vasomotor symptoms Likely	Vasomotor symptoms Most Likely			Increasing symptoms of urogenital atrophy

* Blood draw on cycle days 2-5 ↑ = elevated
** Approximate expected level based on assays using current international pituitary standard

The aging of the reproductive system (ovarian aging) identified in several vertebrate species will lead to the menopause state. Beside the decrease in the follicles numbers, the aging process also plays a role in the menopause state, which is characterized by the decrease in Hypothalamic Pituitary Gonad – Axis function causing irregularity of the estrous cycle. In trial with rats, they had the decreasing of the ovaries function at age of 6 to 18 months characterized by low estrogen levels. This decrease in reproductive system was associated with acute symptoms of menopause including vasomotor disturbances resulting in hot flashes and night sweats, vaginal dryness, depression and mood swings, as well as chronic symptoms including progressive muscle and bone atrophy associated with increasing of susceptibility to osteoporosis, elevation of lipid levels (obesity), and a number of metabolic diseases, such a dyslipidemia, cardiovascular disease, hypertension, and insulin resistance. These problems raise a question:

whether menopause is a consequence of the aging process or endocrine deficiency, or even both.[7,8]

2.3. Role of Activin and Inhibin in Molecular Menopause

The frequency and amplitude of pulsatile GnRH secretion affect the differential synthesis and secretion of FSH and LH, which a slow frequency promotes the FSH synthesis and the elevation of amplitude promotes the LH synthesis. Activin is produced in both pituitary gonadotropes and folliculostellate cell and stimulates the synthesis and secretion of FSH. Inhibin functions as a potent antagonist of activin through separation of activin receptor. Although inhibin is expressed in the pituitary, the gonadal inhibin is a major source of feedback inhibition of FSH.[12]

Inhibins are part of the hypothalamic-pituitary-ovarian axis complex system that is a closed loop negative feedback system. Pituitary gonadotropin secretion is regulated predominantly by inhibins and ovarian steroids.

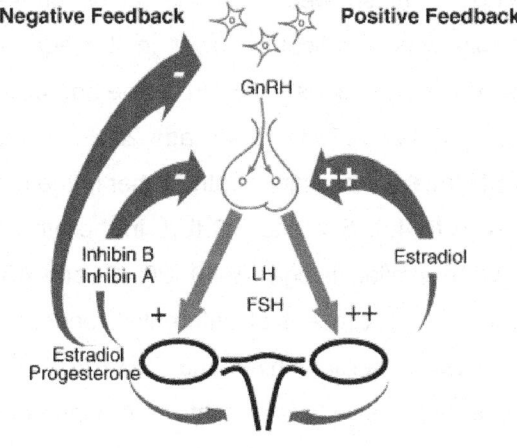

Figure 2. Negative Feedback Mechanism of Inhibin[12]

Inhibin B is a product of the antral follicles granulosa cells, and the levels will decline in line with the decrease in the follicles number concomitant with reproductive aging. The decrease in inhibin B at the end of reproductive age has been shown to trigger a monotropic increase in the FSH follicular phase. The increased FSH, in turn, maintains and sometimes increases E2 production of granulosa cells.[13]

Inhibin was first isolated from the cow's follicular fluid. Inhibins of human cloning as soon as afterwards, were not detected in the postmenopausal women's serum and in the serum of women who have had bilateral oophorectomy. FSH stimulates ovarian inhibin production and then shows a dependent dose stimulation in the follicular phase of menstrual cycle. Both of the inhibin A and inhibin B respond to the exogenous FSH in the follicular phase of the human menstrual cycle.[13]

The immunoreactive inhibin role in reproductive aging was initially explored in the early-follicular (cycle days 4-7) and in the mid-luteal phase (3-12 days before the next menstruation) using serum of women aged 21-49 years as the samples. It showed that the early phase of follicular immunoreactive inhibin was significantly lower in the age of 45-49 years group compared to the younger ones' (128 U/L in the age 45-49 years group compared with 239, 235, and 207 U/L in the age 20-29, 30-39, 40-44 years groups). Average FSH levels were significantly higher in the oldest age group (13,0 IU/L, compared with 4,9; 5,5; and 5,3 IU/L in the other three younger groups). E2 levels were similar in age 45-49, 20-29, and 40-44 years age groups, which supported the concept of differential feedback. A significant negative correlation between serum inhibin and FSH ($r¼\_0.45$, $P <0,05$) was shown, and there was also a significant negative correlation between inhibin and age. With the increasing of age, the FSH levels showed a two-phase linier elevation with an inflection point estimated at about 43 years. The result was consistent with the role of inhibin, in addition to E2, in the FSH regulation during the follicular phase of the menstrual cycle as a function of aging.[13]

Melbourne Women's Midlife Health Project is the first large longitudinal study of the transition experiences of women from the end of the reproductive age until the FMP. The early-follicular phase serum samples showed the decline of inhibin in the early cycle occurred before E2 changed, and while inhibin decreased in the end of the reproductive age, the decrease in E2 was the most significant in the late menopausal transition group (women with amenorrhoea for the last > 3 months). There was a variability marked with FSH, E2 and inhibin consentration in all groups. Including the last transition group, FSH was negatively correlated with E2 (r ¼0.30) and inhibin (r¼_0.39), while inhibin was positively correlated with E2 (r ¼ 0,45). It was concluded that the increase in FSH serum and the decrease in E2 and inhibin were the major endocrine changes associated with menopause transition.[13]

Shortly after the development of specific tests for dimeric inhibin A and B, Klein et al showed that the increase in monotropic FSH levels could be seen in the older women's ovulation associated with the decrease in inhibin B at follicular phase, but not with inhibin A. The measurement of inhibin B was performed on serum samples from the third year Melbourne Women's Midlife Health Project showed a sharp decline in the follicles number and inhibin B in women entering the early menopausal transition, without any changes in E2 or inhibin A. Welt et al also showed that at the follicular phase, inhibin B levels were lower and E2 levels were higher in older women (aged 35-46 years vs aged <35 years). 0,59 data from longitudinal research component showed that the reproductive aging was accompanied by a decrease in both inhibin A and B, and that the decrease in inhibin B was preceded by any decrease in inhibin A or E2 and even might be associated with an increase in E2. They suggested that the loss of inhibin B negative feedback in FSH was the most important factor in increasing the FSH levels by advancing the reproductive age.[13]

Muttikrishna et al studied two groups of women with regular cycles, one with normal FSH levels (<8 IU / L, n=10) and one with an elevation of FSH levels (> 8 IU / L, n= 6), and compared the daily serum hormone levels taken throughout the cycle at a group of young women aged 25-32 years. Older group with high FSH levels had a lower concentration of inhibin B in the early follicular phase and a lower concentration of Inhibin A before the mid-cycle of peaked LH and the mid-luteal phase compared to older women with normal FSH levels. They concluded that the increase in FSH in the early follicular phase in older women was associated with a decrease in inhibin B concentrations in the early follicular phase, and with low concentrations of inhibin A in the luteal phase. Inhibin A is the product of the corpus luteum and play a role in the inhibition of minor gonadotropin secretion. Its function is the hypothalamic-pituitary-ovarian axis has not been clarified.[13]

In a recent study of 77 women classified into STRAW Staging -4, -3, -2, and -1, it was revealed that the ovulatory cycle of FSH, LH, and E2 increased with STRAW development and the progesterone levels decreased in the luteal phase. There are some anovulatory cycles, those are two, zero,one, and nine stages -5 and -4 (n= 21), stages -3 (n= 16), stages -2 (n= 17) and stages -1 (n= 23). By including the anovulatory cycle in the comparative analysis, there was increase in FSH and LH levels in the group, but the increase in E2 was no longer detected. At the early cycle and the average cycle (including ovulation and anovulation), inhibin B levels decreased progressively in the STRAW stage, with the lowest levels detected in the lengthened ovulatory cycles and in the end of menopausal transition period. The inhibin A levels followed by E2 levels, peaked at the peak of E2 and increased during the ovulatory cycle in the STRAW stage.[13]

This study showed that the decrease in Inhibin B and not in Inhibin A was the main factor influencing the elevation of FSH and LH levels concomitantly with increasing in the reproductive age.[13]

Perimenopause refers to the years around menopause in which the function of the ovaries begin to change. The number of ovum decrease and the ovaries become more resistant to the action of Follicle-Stimulating Hormon (FSH), the ovaries begin to reduce the production of estrogen, progesterone, and androgen. The loss of negative feedback mechanism of ovaries estrogen causes the increase in FSH and LH secretion. There is also a decrease in glycoprotein inhibin secretion (selectively inhibits FSH). This action causes a steady FSH elevation which could be a sign that the menopause is imminent.[14]

The changes of hypothalamus rolling at the regular menstrual cycle to be irregular could be experienced by women in two until eight years before the menopause. During that period, the ovarian follicles maturing the ovum will have an accelerated damage so that the number of follicles will run at all. The decrease in inhibin B levels (INH-B) which is a dimeric protein reflexing the decrease in ovarian follicles causes an increase in FSH levels by 20-fold. The early sign of this increase measured at the follicular menstrual cycle is higher than at the female reproductive period, the decrease effect in ovarian steroidal hormones and the elevation in GnRH levels are also increase the LH by 3 to 5-fold.[10]

The decrease in steroidogenesis and Inhibin-A secretion at the luteal phase may cause an increase in FSH levels starting on several days before the menstruation. The determination of this important event is based on data derived from immunoassay FSH. By using the sensitive FSH bioactivity measurement, it is revealed that the increase in FSH bioactivity starting at the mid-end luteal phase.[15]

When a women reached at age of 40s, the anovulatory process began. Before the anovulation occurred more frequently and before the long anovulation occurred, the menstrual cycle lenghtens, starting on 2-8 years before menopause. In a longitudinal study in Australia, if a menstrual cycle is more than 42 days, it is predicted that menopause will be occurred in 1 or 2 years later. This longer menstrual cycle period uniformly precedes the menopause without considering at age when the menses stopped, whether early or late. The main determinant of menstrual cycle length is the duration of follicular phase. This change occurred before the menopause is marked by an elevation of FSH levels and a decrease in inhibin levels, with a normal LH levels and a slight increase in estradiol levels. The length of this cycle is determined by the rate and quality of the follicles' growth and development, and this varies for each woman.[15]

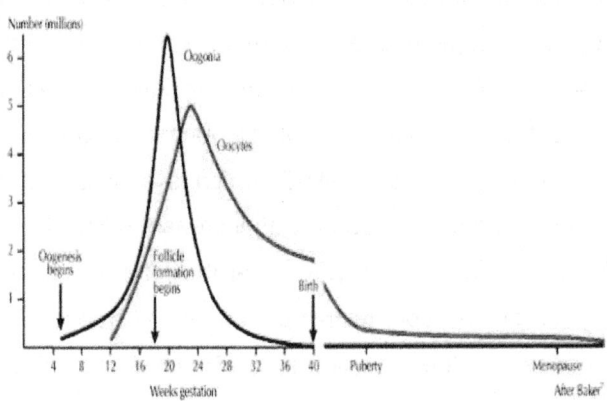

Figure 3. Relationship between Follicles Development[15] and Age[12]

When the rate of follicular reduction began to rise during further reproductive age, but before there was any real changes in menstrual regularity, FSH serum levels begin to rise; LH concentrations remains unchanged. This FSH elevation alone without an increase in LH levels may be a result of age-related changes of the pulsatile GnRH secretion pattern or as a result of progressive follicular reduction and low feedback inhibition rate on FSH pituitary secretion by ovarian hormones. The current evidences support the second explanation. Although the pulsatile GnRH secretion frequency is slower and more stimulates FSH secretion than LH secretion, the frequency and amplitude of the pulsation pattern of LH secretion in the younger or older women is almost similar, even after having an oophorectomy. The inhibin B levels in the circulatory at the luteal phase decrease at or even before the FSH concentration began to rise. There is also a decrease in luteal phase inhibin A serum. Both of the inhibins selectively inhibit FSH pituitary secretion. As a result, FSH levels will rise progressively because of the decline in inhibin production caused by reducing reserved follicles, it could be seen clearly at the early follicular phase. The decreasing inhibin concentration may describe the reduced follicles number, declining of functional follicular capacity in the older follicles, or both. It is observed that the preovulatory follicular fluid inhibin concentration is almost similar in the younger or older women that still have menses, and it is revealed that the most important factor is the number of follicles left.[15]

Along with increasing in age, the FSH levels will rise, the follicular phase is getting shorter but LH levels and luteal phase duration remains unchanged. The menstrual cycle is still regular, but its length and variability decline overall. When the FSH levels rise and the follicular phase is getting shorter, the estradiol levels elevate earlier showing that higher FSH levels rapidly stimulate the follicles development. The earlier estradiol levels elevation is not a result of accelerated follicles growth yet as a result of late follicles development at the initial menstrual cycle and as a result of an earlier dominant follicles selection. The lengths of follicular phase and menstrual cycle reach their lowest limit at about age of 42.[15]

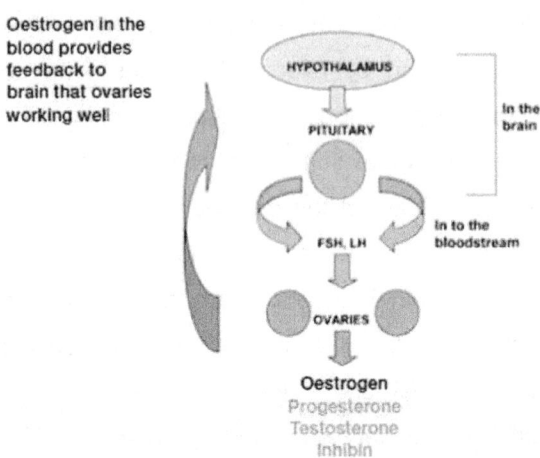

Figure 4. Estrogen Feedback Pathway[16]

Menopause is a gradual process characterized by irregularity of menstruation, ovulation, and ovulatory cycle until the menstruation stops at all. This shows that the molecular pathway controlling the menstrual cycle losses of the ovarian cells. Studies about hormonal status in women showed that menopause was associated with a low levels of estrogen, inhibin, insulin, IGF-I, anti-Mullerian hormone (AMH), and FSH serum.[17]

AMH has been suggested to be a marker of endocrine follicular depletion or ovarian aging. Inhibin is a heterodimeric consists of α and β subunits (inhibin α and β) and is a super family of TGF-β protein. Inhibin β is secreted by the granulosa cells during the early follicular development and recently it has attracted so much attention because of its role in regulating the early follicular development and FSH secretion by the adenopituitary axis. Study carried out in the girls since born to adulthood showed that the inhibin serum levels were lower in age under 6 and peaked between 12 and 18 years when those girls got their menarche.[17]

Observation carried out in the late age women showed that the inhibin serum levels were lower in the women at age of 46-52 compared to those at age 39-45. That study also revealed that in women with menstruation and normal FSH serum levels, there was no difference between the younger and the older groups. The developing findings showed that the abnormality in inhibin secretion (low at serum levels) occurred earlier when the FSH levels were still normal. Indication that the low inhibin serum levels and other intraovarian autocrine and paracrine factors may play a central role in menopause formation. It has been known that the low inhibin levels eliminated the inhibition effect to the pituitary gland, leading to high FSH serum levels.[17]

During the reproductive life of FSH secretion is cyclical, with varying from low to high serum levels; this character maintains the follicular cells sensitivity to FSH. Chronic elevation of FSH and too long contact of ovaries cells to FSH cause receptor to be under regulated and make the follicular cells become no more sensitive to FSH and as a result, there is a defect in final follicular maturation. This might explain about the anovulatory cycle which is a special characteristic of perimenopausal period. Chronic exposure of receptor to ligand has been shown to cause a negative effect to the receptor expression. Why inhibin levels decreased in women approaching menopausal period has not been clarified, there is a possibility that there are local factors secreted by the granulosa cells or oocytes which can regulate inhibin secretion. Factors controlling inhibin secretion during the reproductive life are still controverted; some authors had focused on the possibility of FSH role. Nonetheless, the current relationship between FSH and inhibin during perimenopausal and menopausal period is not very supportive the FSH role in regulation of inhibin secretion. In the menopausal period, low inhibin serum levels occur when FSH serum levels are normal and they remain unchanged even after menopause period has come when FSH serum levels are high, and it indicates that besides FSH, there is another factor responsible for inhibin secretion regulation.[17]

Former studies had shown that there was local factor such as insulin growth factor-1 (IGF-1) in controlling inhibin secretion. During reproductive phase, studies showed that IGF-1 stated in the endometrial cells and ovarian tissues increased the granulose cells secretion and steroidal hormones secretion. Another study showed that in reaching the menopausal period, IGF-1 decreased in the ovarian tissues, and was followed by gradual decrease in inhibin B serum levels. Low IGF-1 levels has also been reported in endometrium of postmenopausal women. Therefore, it is suggested that IGF-1 might be role as a paracrine factor increasing inhibin B secretion during reproductive phase and decrease in IGF-I in the ovarian tissues can lead to the fail of inhibin secretion by granulose cells. It has been known that oocytes played a key role in controlling its function by influencing follicular cells function.[17]

The actual estimation of female ovarian primordial follicles in some variation of age derives from histological preparat analysis. Mathematical model has been suggested for years to describe the relationship between non-growing follicles (NGFs) and age. Faddy et al. in 1992 concluded that the oocytes decline rates followed biphasic pattern with decelerated rate occurred at age about 37,5 years. Recently, Hansen et al. revealed that the decline in ovarian follicles number was associated with the increase of age. In a recent study conducted by Kelsey et al. in 2012, it is showed that AMH serum levels positively correlated with NGFs in women aged 5-51 years. Data analysis of Kelsey et al. was based on systematical data aggregation of 8 studies, where the population's NGFs had been extrapolated from the number of stereological manual NGF of small subset ovarian tissues, and 25 cohort studies reported normative AMH levels in limited age ranging. Overall, those data supported that AMH serum could be used as another ovarian marker.

Moreover, our data showed that mother menopausal age categories could predict the decrease levels of reserved ovarian.[18]

Clearly, our data couldn't explain whether mother menopausal age is a direct predictor to the menopausal age or to the possibility to get pregnant. Nevertheless, from biological side, it is logic to assume that low reserved ovarian had longlasting effect that might shorten the reproductive phase. Therefore, we assumed that a marker such as "menopausal age" combined with AMH or AFC, and age chronologist might be a more complete figure to evaluate individual's reserved ovarian.[18]

2.4. Clinical Manifestation of Menopause

Problems frequently complained within this period include irritability, depression, fatigue, lack of enthusiasm, insomnia, hot flashes, sweating, chilling, and headache. When a woman enters menopause, physical discomforts such as stiffnes and pain could occur suddenly in the whole body. This stiffness is sometimes accompanied by a feeling of heat or cold, dizziness, headache, fatigue, restless, irritable, and palpitations. After menopause, women will experience senile period. At this time, they reach a new hormonal balance so that there is no more vegetative or psychological disorders.[7-9,19]

Several symptoms women experienced are associated with the increase in age and the decrease in ovarian activity. The other symptoms might be generally related with aging. Evidences showed a link to menopause described in this following symptoms:[20]

- Hot flashes and night sweats (also called vasomotor symptoms, because of vascular dilation)

- Vaginal dryness, that can cause a painful sexual intercourse. Some women also have memory problems. This may be related to estrogen changes during transitional period.

It can be reassured that these following symptoms are caused or not by menopause, other factors come along with aging, or combination of menopause and aging:[20]

- Incontinence
- Physical complaints such as fatigue, stiffness, or joint pain
- Mood swings such as depression, agitation, and irritability. And symptoms similar in premenstrual syndrome.

The experts gathered at NIH State-of-the-Science conference noted that menopause is a normal part of a woman aging and suggested that a menopause should not be considered as a "medical disorders" (or seen as a disease).[20]

2.5. Osteoporosis in Menopausal Women

Nowadays, the increase in human life expectancy rates will rise the degenerative disease prevalence, and it is estimated that until 2025, there will be an increase in osteoporosis number. Osteoporosis is most commonly found in late age postmenopausal women.

Menopause is the cessation of menstruation permanently as a result of unactive ovarian follicles. The decrease in ovarian function causes decline in sexual hormones production, estrogen and progesterone. This will affect the cyclic activity of hypothalamus and pituitary. In the end, it will cause neurologic and metabolic disorders clinically appeared as perimenopausal symptoms. The most common problem complained is the bone symptom.

Osteoporosis is the main problem in menopausal women. More than 10 million of Americans people have osteoporosis and more than 34 million people have low bone density that increases the risk of osteoporosis and fractures. Bone will always do remodeling every year. the changes in bone size and shape are based on epiphyseal closure at the end of puberty followed by consolidation period for 5-10 years.[14]

Bone is a living tissue with a dynamic structure that can adapt and do remodelling. Its functions are very extensive, starting with forming a strong skeleton, muscle and organ protection, source of hematopoiesis, and playing a role in maintaining metabolic balance of minerals serum, especially for calcium and phosphate. Bone is composed of cells, matrix, protein, and mineral deposit. It has three basic cells- osteoblasts, osteocytes, and osteoclasts. Osteoblasts are bone-forming cells derived from osteoid and bone mineral matrix. A complete process is characterized by osteoblast reforming into osteocytes and trapped in the bone matrix containing minerals. Osteoclasts are resorptive to bone during the growth period and remodel the bones by secreting lactic acid and collagenase that destroy the bone minerals and collagen.[15]

Remodelling is determined by homeostasis od osteoblasts and osteoclasts. Until age of 50, osteoclasts have the same level of activity as osteoblasts. Age induced osteoporosis occurs in age of 60 and over, and menopause induced osteoporosis occurs in age of 50 and over. Remodeling rate is about 2-10% of skeleton mass each year. This process is affected by some factors, such as local factor causing a series of events on the Activation-Resorption-Formation (ARF) concept. This process is influenced by mitogenic proteins derived from bones stimulating proteoblast to cleave and reform into osteoblasts as a result of resorption activity of osteoclasts. Another factor affecting this process is hormonal factor. Remodeling process will be rise by parathyroid hormones, growth hormones, and 1,25 $(OH)_2$

vitamin D. While those inhibiting the remodeling process are calcitonin, estrogen, and glucocorticoid. These process interferes with bone remodeling, and causing osteoporosis.[16]

Osteoporosis is occurred because the number and activity of osteoclasts is more predominant than the number and activity of osteoblasts, so that the decrease in bone density occurred. Related with menopause, this event is caused by estrogen deficiency and stress.[17]

Estrogen is a hormone that plays a key role in bone metabolism because of its influence in osteoblasts and osteoclasts activities. Osteoblast have α and β estrogen receptor in the cytosol.

The decrease in estrogen levels will directly cause an increase in proinflammatory cytokines such as IL-1, IL-3, IL-6, LIF (Leukemia Inhibiton Factor), oncostatin M, Ciliary Neutropic Factor, GM-CSF (Granulocyte-macrophage Colony Stimulating Factor), M-CF, RANK-L (receptor activator of nuclear factor-κB ligand), and TNF-α which have a role in triggering osteoclasts in osteoclastogenesis process. RANKL is synthesized by osteoblasts and stromal cells expressed by osteoclast progenitor cells in the bone marrow to induce osteoclastogenesis. Osteoprotegerin is synthesized by osteoblasts and stromal cells as inhibitor of RANKL receptors to prevent linking between RANKL with RANK (receptor activator of nuclear factor-κB). RANK-L will induce the JNK1 (Jun N-terminal Kinase 1) activity and osteoclastogenic activator protein-1, c-fos, and c-jun so that the monocytes could differentiate into osteoclasts rapidly. Int the other hand, osteoblastic stromal cells have expression on the surface of RANK-L that will be linked to RANK on the osteoclast progenitor surface to stimulate the differentiation of osteoclast cells.[18]

Indirectly, a decrease in estrogen also causes the decline in osteoprotegrin and TGF-β (Transforming Growth Factor beta) in the osteoblastic and stromal cells mediating osteoblasts to repair the destructive bone area and to increase osteoclast apoptosis. Wnt signaling that is important in osteoblast formation is reduced because of LRP5 gen (LDL Receptor-Related. Protein 5) which is not too sensitive in the menopausal period.[19]

In the level of bone density and quality, there is a microarchitectural element disruption of trabecular bones, periosteal envelop expansion, endocortical trabecularization, and declining in bone elements mineralization. There is a significant relationship between low bone density and fracture risk. The most common fracture occurred is pelvic, vertebrae, and extremities fracture. Mostly 50% of the population experienced these can not live a normal life any more.[20]

The purpose of osteoporosis therapy is to prevent fracture by increasing the bone strength and reducing the risk to fall and get trauma, minimizing the symptoms because of fracture and skeletal deformity, and maximizing the physical function.[20,21]

Pharmacological therapy indications:[21]

- Pelvic or vertebrae fracture
- T-score under -2,5 of vertebrae, femur and pelvic
- T scores between -1 to -2.5 for 10 years risk of fracture were assessed with FRAX tool

Pharmacological therapy:[21]

1. Bisphosphonates

    Bisphosphonates is the most widely used drugs for osteoporosis treatment. Bisphosphonates was taken on a empty stomach condition in the morning with a glass of water. Even though the absorption rate of bisphosphonates is just below <1%, but still useful for osteoporosis.

Bisphosphonates intravenous may be given but with the elevating risk of hypersensitvity for 30-40%.[21]

a. Alendronate

Alendronate approved dose is 10 mg each days or 70 mg each weeks. Alendronate has showed a decreased risk fracture of spine, pelvis, and os non-vetebra. Alendronate increases bone density after 4 – 5 years of using its drug.[21]

b. Risedronate

Risedronate approved dose is 5 mg each days or 35 mg per weeks. Risedronate slightly decreased the acceleration of losing bone after 3 years therapy.[21]

c. Ibandronate

Ibandronate approved dose is 2.5 mg each days for 5 years using its drug. The effects of its drug are decreasing the losing of bone density and increasing bone density.[21]

d. Zolendronate acid

Zolendronate acid approved dose is 5 mg each days for the same effect with others bisphophonates.[21]

2. Calcium Supplementation

The absorption of calcium slightly decreased with increasing age because the reduction of an active vitamin D biologically and having a significant disruption after menopause. A positive calcium balance compulsory for achieving an adequate prevention for osteoporosis. Calcium supplementation (1.000 mg each days) decreasing the losing of bone and decreasing of bone fracture, especially the person who is having a low diet of calcium.[21]

The average woman takes 500 mg calcium on its diet, so the supplement for each days is equal with an additional 500 mg. Woman who didn't undergo estrogen therapy needs a supplement at least 1.000 mg each days to gain a 1.500 mg each days diet reccomendation. Woman who has a calcium supplements for more that 500 mg each days should undergo a calcium and phosphor blood levels test within first 2 years. If it's normal, than there is no need further observation.[21]

Estrogen acts to improve calcium absorbtion (with increasing a 1,25-dihydroxyvitamin D levels) and may lowering an active calcium supplement dose. In order to remain a zero calcium balances, woman who has estrogen therapy need 1.000 mg calcium supplements total each days.[21]

Estrogen acts to improve calcium absorption and have a calcium supplement in an effective dose without the side effect because the higher dose (constipation and flatulence). We must confim, even though calcium supplement is important but we cannot achieve the same protection as hormonal osteoporosis. But still, the advantages of estrogen on spine is decreased wihout a calcium supplementation.[21]

The calcium supplementation is more important in adolescent rather than in reproductive years (when a bone forming is minimal). Increasing diet of calcium in adolescent give a significant increasing of bone density and skeletal mass that give a protection for osteoporosis in later life. under 25 years, for years accumulation of bone, calcium diet each days shoul be 1.500 mg. This amount was recommended for pregnancy and breastfeed. Most of the calcium came from milk production; relying on others food is not easy/simple because the higher needed on the others food to have the exactly the amount of calcium as normal milk each days.[21]

There are dozens calcium supplement in market, that has a calcium carbonate, calcium lactate, calcium phosphate, calcium gluconate. Calcium carbonate tablet is the cheapest and has most of calcium elemental. (40%). Calcium lactate has 13% of calcium, calcium citric has 23% and calcium gluconate has just 9%. The most efficient calcium supplementation occurs when a single dose that no more than 500 mg and taken during night.[21]

3. Raloxifene

FDA approved raloxifene for prevention and treatment on osteoporosis post menopausal. Raloxifene oral may be given while eating and there is no provision of advice to use like biphosphonate.[21]

4. Teriparatide

This medicine/drug are recombinants of PTH(1-34) 20 microgram per subcutaneous injection.. Teriparatide increases bone density and decreases bone destruction. Efficacy was acquired after 2 years.[21]

5. Calcitonin

Calcitonin approved dose is 200 IU spray or injection. There is no studies to assess how long calcitonin must be given to decrease risk of bone fracture.[21]

6. Denosumab

This medicine/drug is monoclonal antibody RANKLS that decrease amount of RANKL on micromolecular of bone, decrease precursor cell differentiation to mature osteoclast, and decrease the function and survival of osteclast. The approved dose is 60 mg subcutaneous injection every 6 months.[21]

7. Estrogen

Althogh estrogen regarded as drug of choice for osteoporosis in post menopause, FDA never approved estrogen for this. Dose that frequently used is 0.625 mg each days. estrogen conjugated quine with or without medroxyprogesterone acetate to increase bone density especially on spine, spine, shoulder. Actual indication for estrogen use is perimenopausal symptoms. This is because, if estrogen delivery was stopped, the protective effect of osteoporosis was also stopped.[21]

There is no studies that shows the advantages of using the combination couples drugs for osteoprorosis postmenopausal threapy.[21,22]

8. Sports

Sprots exercises can strengthen our bones. By doing sport exercise regularly and correctly for 30 minutes a days and 3 days a week, It will be useful in the preventive and treatment of osteoporosis, will increase mineral content of bone in elderly women. To be effective, exercise must exert a load on the bones, especially the spine. Regular runs will not be enough. However, fast walking can slow bone loss in the pelvis.[21]

There is useful activity like running, weight training, aerobics, climbing stairs and sports other than swimming. The effect of weight bearing exercise on bone density are additive when combine with hormone therapy. Although regular walking has a small impact on bone density, but still it is reasonable to have a beneficial effect upon the risk fracture. These changes plus the sport itself will improve balance and reduce the risk of falls. For this reason, walking, even after adjustments for bone density and weight are associated with reducing risk of pelvic fracture.[21]

2.6. Menopause Rating Scale (MRS)

Menopause Rating Scale (MRS) is a scale of quality of life that was developed in early 90s to assess the severity of menopausal complaints as a response to the lack of a standarized scale to measure the severity of the symptoms of aging and its effects on quality of life. Validation of MRS began several years ago with the goal to establish a tool for measuring quality of life, which can easily be filled. The purpose of making MRS is (1) to allow comparisons among women with different conditions, (2) to compare the severity of disease in a certain time interval, and (3) to measure the changes that occurs before and after treatment. MRS scale have formally standarized rule-based psychometric and for the first time MRS scale was publish in Germany. Three separate dimension has been identified, which explains 59% of total variance found (factor analysis) : psychological, somato vegetative, and urogenital subscales. MRS scale consists of 11 items (symptoms or complaints). Each symptom that contained in the scale can be assigned a value of 0 (no symptoms) to 4 (severe symptoms) depending on the level of symptoms obtained after the woman fills the question of scale (checking the appropriate box). The assessment is basically simple, for example : the score will increase along with the increasing severity of subjectivity symptoms which is obtained from each item (score 0 : no symptoms, a score 4 : symptoms very severe). Respondent by itself will show his own preseption by checking 1 of the 5 possibilities box that available for each item. [7]

Currently, MRS scale was accepted in international. First, this scale was translated into English, which is followed by a translation into another language. The latest international methodologies reccomendation is also included. This time the scale is available in several language : Brazil, England, France, Germany, Indonesia, Italy, Mexico/Argentina, Spain, Sweden, and Turkey.[7]

Yang manakah dari gejala-gejala yang tertera di bawah ini yang Anda alami sekarang ini dan seberapa berat atau ringankan gejala-gejala tersebut?
Tolong Anda berikan tanda 'X' di kotak yang tepat untuk setiap gejala yang tertera di bawah ini. Untuk gejala-gejala yang sekarang ini tidak Anda alami, berikan tanda 'X' di kotak nomor '0'.

	tidak ada	ringan	menengah	berat	sangat berat
	0	1	2	3	4
1. Badan terasa sangat panas, berkeringat	☐	☐	☐	☐	☐
2. Rasa tidak nyaman pada jantung (detak jantung yan tidak biasa, jantung berdebar)	☐	☐	☐	☐	☐
3. Masalah tidur (susah tidur, susah untuk tidur nyenyak, bangun terlalu pagi)	☐	☐	☐	☐	☐
4. Perasaan tertekan (merasa tertekan, sedih, mudah menangis, tidak bergairah/lesu, mood yang berubah-ubah)	☐	☐	☐	☐	☐
5. Mudah marah (merasa gugup, rasa marah, agresif)	☐	☐	☐	☐	☐
6. Rasa resah (rasa gelisah, rasa panik)	☐	☐	☐	☐	☐
7. Kelelahan fisik dan mental (menurunnya kinerja secara umum, berkurangnya daya ingat, menurunnya konsentrasi, mudah lupa/pikun)	☐	☐	☐	☐	☐
8. Masalah-masalah seksual (perubahan dalam gairah seksual, aktifitas seksual dan kepuasan seksual)	☐	☐	☐	☐	☐
9. Masalah-masalah pada kandung dan saluran kemih (sulit buang air kecil, sering buang air kecil, buang air kecil yang tidak terkontrol)	☐	☐	☐	☐	☐
10. Kekeringan pada vagina (rasa kering atau terbakar, pada vagina, kesulitan dalam berhubungan intim)	☐	☐	☐	☐	☐
11. Rasa tidak nyaman pada persendian dan otot (sakit pada persendian, kelhan rematik)	☐	☐	☐	☐	☐

Figure 5 . Menopause Rating Scale[7]

Caption: [7]

Scores for level/degree of severity of the complaint based on subscales are as follows:

• Total Score 22 - None, a bit: 0-4; mild: 5-8; moderate: 9-16; severe: 17+

CHAPTER 3

GENERAL MANAGEMENT OF MENOPAUSAL WOMEN AND ROLE OF TESTOSTERONE IN MENOPAUSE

3.1. General Management Of Menopausal Women

For decades, hormone therapy is mostly used for the treatment of menopausal symptoms. Estrogen has been used as menopausal hormone therapy in women whose uterus has been removed. Progestin, a synthetic form of estrogen-progesterone related called, combined with estrogen in menopausal hormone therapy in women who still have their uterus. Progestin stops the growth of cells in the lining of the uterus. Continued growth of these cells can lead to cervical cancer.[20]

Women's Health Initiative (WHI), a 15-year research program was launched in 1991, was designed to resolve most common causes of death, disability, and poor quality of life in postmenopausal women. Research program to test the effectiveness of hormone replacement therapy in women, who at the time was considered a promising intervention. The findings from two clinical trials WHI checked:[20]

- The use of estrogen plus progestin in women with a uterus
- The use of estrogen in women without a uterus only.

HRT (combined estrogen-progesterone to women with intact uterus, and estrogen for those who have had a hysterectomy) is very effective, reducing hot flashes and other menopausal symptoms 80% to 90% of the reporting period. But the widely publicized Women's Health Initiative of increased risk of breast cancer, coronary heart disease, stroke, and venous thromboembolism in women receiving estrogen and progesterone to encourage patients to tappering off HRT, or decline to start it. Initial reports of the last decade, however, and further analysis and additional studies have found that for some women, and under some circumstances, HRT may, in fact, safe and effective.[21]

Age and time of menopause is a key criteria. For women who aged <60 years and within 10 years of the onset of menopause, HRT appears to be a safe short-term treatment. While probably the most significant risk after 10 years of use, doctors should try to limit the HRT whenever possible.[21]

Women were ≥ 60 years and those at high risk for cardiovascular disease or breast cancer, or both, should not take HRT. When recipe HRT to patients without contraindications, there are things you can do to minimize risk:[21]

- Limit the duration of HRT to shorten the required treatment.
- Use the transdermal delivery system. Compared with oral administration, patches appear to reduce the risk of thromboembolism
- Recipe a low dose regimens of HRT. Low doses can reduce the risk of cardiovascular disease, but it usually will take longer to relieve symptoms, 8 to 12 weeks versus 4 weeks for women in the standard dose. A low-dose regimen is very important for women who are obese. Because estradiol levels serum were higher in this patient population, they need a smaller quantity of estrogen and progesterone to achieve cure symptoms.
- Lower slowly over 6 to 12 months which can minimize the severity and frequency of hot flashes.

Hormone compounds. Some women prefer a hormone, based on the results of blood or saliva test individually, in the hope avoiding risks associated with HRT. While the compound is usually marketed safer and more effective in reducing the symptoms of menopause, however, there is limited evidence of their success. What else, the lack of standardization, so that variations in formulation and dosage from one product to another, raising questions about the safety of hormonal compounds.[21]

Both selective serotonin reuptake inhibitors (SSRIs) and serotonin-norepinephrine reuptake inhibitors (SNRIs), which targets the neurotransmitter involved in the hypothalamic thermoregulatory center, has been found to reduce both the severity and frequency of hot flashes. Women who have hot flashes have a 2 times increase in risk for depression, and antidepressant therapy can help ease mood disorders in addition to providing relief of vasomotor symptoms, even in women who do not meet the criteria for clinical depression.

Venlafaxine, desvenlafaxine, and paroxetine have been shown to provide relief of best vasomotor symptoms, with a reduction in symptoms of 67% vs 15% with placebo. It is important to note, however, that the study each agent has a different inclusion criteria and randomization different meanings.[21]

Certain antihypertensives (clonidine and methyldopa) and antiepileptic gabapentin may reduce hot flashes, but not the optimal treatment. Clonidine has been shown to be effective both oral and transdermal forms, but these drugs are associated with hypotension, among other adverse effects Methyldopa not been well studied and not seen as a first-line agent and, although gabapentin at doses ≥ 900 mg / day reduced the frequency of hot flashes, many women can not tolerate the nausea, headache, dizziness, confusion are common, and other adverse effects.[21]

Little research has found that specific activity, such as respiration pacing and yoga, increase hot flashes, but larger studies are needed to clarify the big effect. Lifestyle interventions, such as limiting alcohol consumption, reducing the intake of spicy food, avoid hot drinks, and eliminate caffeine, can reduce hot flashes as well.[21]

3.2. Role Of Testosterone In Menopause

Testosterone is one type of steroid hormones. He is the main androgenic hormone produced by the interstitial cells (Leydig) in response to LH stimulation of the anterior pituitary gland. Androgens are steroid hormones with 19 atom C. This hormone has a molecular weight of 288.41 Dalton and dominant in men (Koolman, 2005. Murray, 2003).

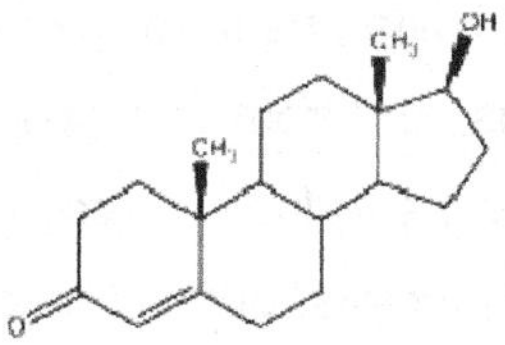

Figure 6. Chemical Structure of Testosterone[22]

Androgens and sex hormone are produced by the ovaries and adrenal glands in females and testes by men. The main androgen hormones in women are adrenal androgens and testosterone. In women 50% of testosterone is produced by the ovaries and adrenal glands are directly released into blood.[23]

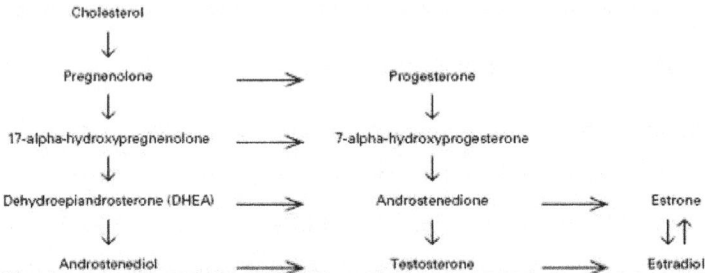

Figure 7. Synthesis of Testosterone[23]

The production of testosterone in women is derived from three sources: the ovaries, adrenal glands, and from changes in the peripheral circulation of androgen. Testosterone levels reduce in accordance aging. This decrease is related to a combination of factors: production of androgens from the adrenal glands progressively decrease as aging, although the production of testosterone from the ovary is usually intact after menopause, adrenal secretion against androstenedione decreased by approximately 50%. Lower androstenedione causes a significant decrease in testosterone in peripheral changes to the current menopause.[24]

The cells that produce steroid hormones in the ovaries do not store steroid but produce these hormones due to the effect of LH and FSH during the normal menstrual cycle. Step-by-step process and the enzymes involved in the synthesis of steroid hormones as well as the similarities found in the ovaries, adrenals, and testes. However, special enzymes needed to catalyze specific steps divided separately and probably not many or even not present in all cell types. During the process of development of ovarian follicles, estrogen synthesis of cholesterol requires tight integration between the theca cells and granulosa cells are sometimes referred to as the two cell steroidogenesis (Fig. 2.7). FSH receptor confined to granulosa cells, whereas the LH receptor is limited to the theca cells to the final stage of follicular development, while later also found in granulosa cells. Theca cells located around the follicle has a high vascularity and use of cholesterol, especially those derived from circulating lipoproteins, as an initial starting point of the synthesis of androstenedione and testosterone under the influence of LH. Androstenedione and testosterone to move across the basal lamina to the granulosa cells, which do not receive direct blood supply. Mural granulosa cells are very rich in aromatase and be under the influence of FSH to produce estradiol, which is the main steroid secreted during ovarian follicular phase and is the most potent estrogen. Androstenedione produced by the theca cells and testosterone are also secreted into the peripheral blood cells which can then be converted into dihydrotestosterone in the skin and into estrogens in adipose tissue. Interstitial cells of ovarian hilum is functionally similar to the Leydig cells and also able to secrete androgen.

Biological data support an important physiological effects of testosterone in women. Testosterone act directly via androgen receptors throughout the body, including in the areas of the brain, particularly the hypothalamus and amygdala; and peripheral side including bone, breast, skin, skeletal muscle, adipose, vascular, and genital tissues. The effects mediated by aromatization of testosterone to estrogen as hormone androgen is an essential precursor for the biosynthesis of estrogen on ekstragonad and ovarian tissue.

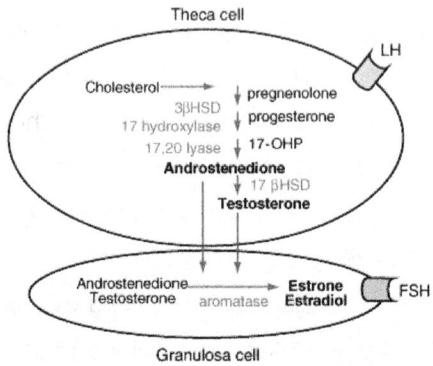

Figure 8. The Mechanism of *Two-Cell Model for Steroidogenesis*[12]

Imbalance biosynthesis or metabolism of androgens in women may have an unpleasant effect on the whole system. Testosterone, estrogen may affect sexual arousal, bone mineral density, muscle mass, adipose tissue distribution, Moog, energy, and ability to live physiology.[26]

In young women, testosterone is made by the ovaries along with estrogen and progesterone. Testosterone is also produced by other tissues such as skin and body fat by converting a hormone produced by the adrenal gland called dehydroepiandrosterone (DHEA) and DHEA sulfate (DHEAS) and androstenedione from ovarium.[23]

Ovaries make estrogen by converting testosterone into estrogen. After menopause, when the ovaries are not able to do its job, the fat tissue of women become the main source of estrogen that are made by converting adrenal androgens into estrogens in adipose tissue. Testosterone and other related hormones in the body (DHEA/DHEAS) are important for female physiology.[23]

Estrogen is made of testosterone and other adrenal hormones your body is not able to make testosterone and estrogen. Therefore important rules of testosterone to provide the basic structure of the production of estrogen. Testosterone has a direct effect on the free androgen receptors in various parts of the body, and some women may experience a variety of symptoms associated with testosterone action.[23]

There is few free testosterone in the blood circulation. As many as 60 % of testosterone bound protein known as sex hormone binding globulin (SHBG) and 33 % bound to the blood protein called albumin. Therefore only 1-2 % of testosterone in the blood circulation in young women who are bound in blood or free in the blood.[23]

This pathway is important to know the advantages and disadvantages of testosterone in the blood:[23]

1. Low SHB indicates that more testosterone in circulation so that women with lower SHBG looks more masculine with bushy hair or acne.
2. SHBG increased free testosterone signaling least. Estrogen therapy, either as oral contraceptives or hormone therapy increases SHBG, causing a decrease in free testosterone and can cause a decrease in sexual desire and libido as a side effect.

Aging affects women androgen production by two different mechanisms :[23]

1. Increasing age and adrenal glands cause a decline in DHEA and DHEAS progressively important as a source of estrogen and testosterone in women .
2. Testosterone levels decline with increasing age associated with reduced ovarian production and reduced adrenal function . The fall in the value of testosterone slowly before menopause; and testosterone levels did not change during menopause.

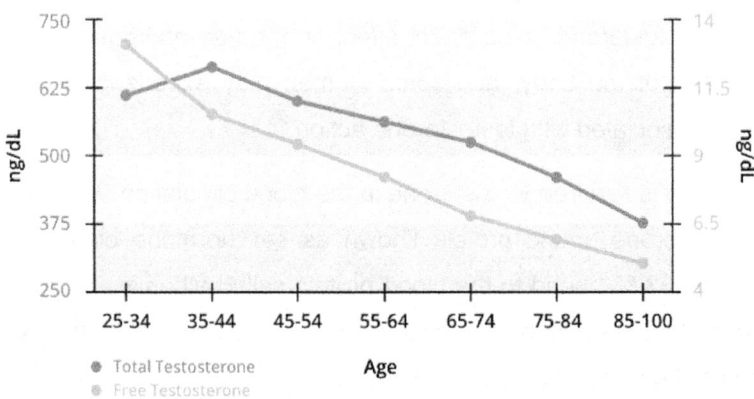

Figure 9. The Decrease in Testosterone Levels Along with Age[25]

Total testosterone was measured directly, radioimunoassay method clinically useful in the study population of low testosterone in women. Free testosterone is calculated using equation Sodergard. Estimates of free testosterone has been shown to have a strong correlation with dialiasis equilibrium, which is generally accurate method of measurement of free testosterone. The results showed a decrease in total and free testosterone, dehydroepiandrosterone (DHEAS), and androstenedione by age, starting mid aged 30 years.[26]

Testosterone may work with many different roads on the network but is an area that requires further investigation. The main action of testosterone seems directly via the androgen receptor (AR). However, testosterone is an important precursor for the production of estradiol in the target tissue. So that the action of testosterone may result in changes to estradiol, and in the genome via the estrogen receptor (ER) beta and alpha, or non genome via estrogenic mechanisms. Grohe et.al. reported an elegant experiment that shows biosynthesis estrogen from testosterone in cardiac myocytes and activation of ER alpha and beta and downstream gene targets.[27]

Biological data support important physiological effects of testosterone in women. Testosterone acts directly via androgen receptors throughout the body, including in areas such as the brain, particularly the hypothalamus and amygdala; and at peripheral sites including bone, breast, skin, skeletal muscle, and adipose, vascular, and genital tissues.[28]

3.3. Use of Testosterone in Menopausal Hormone Therapy

Although postoperative menopausal women may be the group most likely to benefit from testosterone therapy, women with natural menopause are equally likely to benefit. Women who experience premature ovarian failure, especially secondary chemotherapy or radiotherapy, also should be considered for therapy testosteron.[29]

Examination of physical factors, psychological, cultural, and sexual relations affect the well-being and sexual function. Therefore, women who experience a decrease in sexual interest with or without interruption of sexual response should be assessed for psychological health, physical, and social in general. Stress , fatigue, relationship problems, depression, and common side effects of treatment contribute to a reduced sexual interest. Medical conditions that can cause fatigue and low welfare, such as iron deficiency and hypothyroidism, should be removed. While the presence of factors and conditions should not exclude women from testosterone treatment, they must be managed simultaneously.[29]

Sex hormones exert both organizational and activational effects, which are relevant to sexual function, and their actions are mediated by non-genomic as well as direct and indirect genomic pathways. Research data suggest that sex hormones (estrogen, androgens and even progesterone) prime the brain to be selectively responsive to sexual incentives inducing a neurochemical state favourable to sexual response. When an imbalance occurs between the dopaminergic system, which increases sexual desire and excitement, and norepinephrine system, which affects arousal and orgasm, women may feel unable to begin the sexual response cycle. In addition, an overactive serotoninergic system can decrease desire and delay orgasm. Situational variables, such as stress and fatigue, and/or pharmacological compounds (i.e. selective serotonin reuptake inhibitors [SSRIs]) may tonically activate endogenous inhibitory mechanisms. Alternatively, some metabolic and/or hormonal conditions (i.e. menopause) may endogenously blunt sexual excitatory mechanisms. The net balance between stimulatory and inhibitory factors brings about the ability to experience sexual desire. Other mediators have been postulated to play a critical role in women's sexuality, including oxytocin, melanocortins, opioid and endocannabinoid systems.[30]

There are multiple ways in which androgens target the brain regions (hypothalamic, limbic and cortical) involved in sexual function and behaviour. T directly or throughout aromatization to E2 contributes to the initiation of sexual activity and permission for sexual behaviour in multiple areas of the brain.[34] A further non-genomic action by T metabolites on sexual receptivity has been described at the hypothalamic level. On the other hand, the brain is a steroidogenic organ itself and it is capable of producing from precursors and/or *de novo* its own neurosteroids relevant to sexual pathways. The concept of intracrinology has to be taken into account because this local production seems to be more critical to women's sexual desire and function than peripheral androgens. Indeed, circulating levels of sex hormones may not reflect biological activity within the target tissues and other metabolites, either within the cells or released into the plasma, may be even more important to drive sexual interest.[16] Finally, it is worth remembering that every woman possesses her own threshold of tissue responsiveness to hormonal variation depending on several factors, from genetic disposition and age to lifestyle and personal experiences, and a wide range of individual responses may be observed at physical and behavioural level in basal conditions and following hormonal manipulations.[30]

The approved testosterone needs formulated for women is clear. Women in America are looking for testosterone therapy, and gynecologist support them with good recipe testosterone cream and testosterone troches or products that provide the right dosage for male testosterone replacement.[29]

Either oral undecanoate testosterone or methyltestosterone can be given to women, because they can effect lipid levels, and testosterone undecanoate can cause insulin resistance. The available data indicate that the most physiological is parenteral testosterone, especially with transdermal formulations.[29]

Doctors have given women testosterone for decades. Testosterone treated women experienced improvement in symptoms and improved the welfare of the common sexually if want to continue therapy. Randomized controlled trial have shown the efficacy of testosterone therapy compared with placebo for several parameters of sexual function. Other effects of testosterone therapy may be beneficial, such as reduced risk of fractures and a beneficial effect on cognitive function and cardiovascular function, require further investigation.[29]

When considering starting testosterone treatment, only the dose the right one for women to be prescribed. Women should be fully informed that although the combined findings from randomized trials of testosterone conducted to date have not shown an increased risk of breast cancer or cardiovascular disease, the evidence is not yet available on the safety of long term testosterone administration.[29]

Methyltestosterone, synthetic testosterone, combined with estrogen ester is allowed by FDA for use in women. This product is commercially known as Estraest (Abbot Laboraories) and Estratest HS (Abbott Laboratories), although only a generic version is available at this time. Bioidentical Testosterone is not allowed FDA for using in women.[5,32]

The use of testosterone in women is most often considered in postmenopausal women, while women have symptoms such as reduced sense of comfort, low libido, unexplained fatigue, decreased muscle strength, and changes in cognition or memory, all sof this called "female androgen insufficiency". Several studies have shown that testosterone insufficiency resulted in low women sexual stimulation. Offer positive effect including improvement of sexual function, mood, pour density, and a skinny body. Although the data are limited, the addition of testosterone than estrogen in postmenopausal women resulted in a positive effect on sexual arousal. Data are inadequate to strengthen the use of testosterone to improve the symptoms of menopause, feeling comfortable, secure bone, or cognition.[32]

Long-term effects on the breast is unknown. Epidemiological studies of exogenous testosterone on cardiovascular disease in women is still not conducted. There is no relationship between exogenous testosterone and hypertension, arterial vascular reactivity, blood viscosity, or hypercoagulability has been reported. Potential risks of testosterone include acne, hair and face excessive body (4% to 6%), deep voice, weight gain, emotional instability, and lipid profile shift. In addition, oral methyltestosteron may decrease high-density lipoprotein cholesterol, increasing the hematocrit value, causing abnormalities in liver function tests, and may cause toxicity 3 of 100,000 people per year.

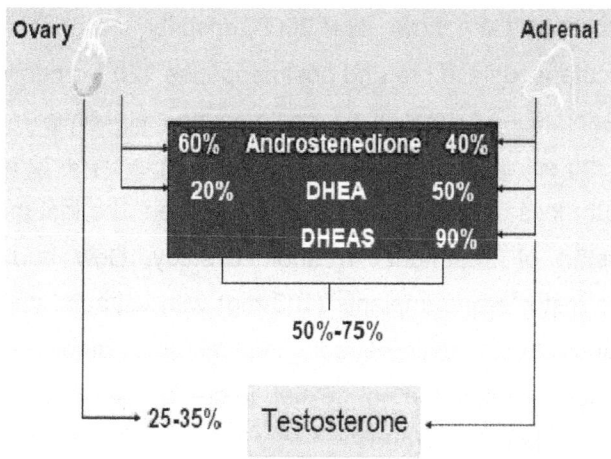

Figure 10. Androgen Productions in Premenopausal Women.[33]

Testosterone therapy in women requires careful consideration and per individual. Testosterone therapy may be considered for women of estrogen due to the lack of data for the use of testosterone in postmenopouse women who do not get a estrogen therapy. Decision use of testosterone, adding additional preparation is often conducted to choose methyltestosterone because it will increase the risk of hepatotoxicity and lipid effects are not pleasant.[32]

Preliminary research finds positive effects of testosterone implants on estrogen replacement therapy in postmenopausal women who have lost their libido. Studd et al showed 136 of 300 women (43.5%) came to the clinic complaining about loss of libido, one of the three major problems. Women are persistent loss of libido, even if it had been given oral estrogen (conjugated equine estrogens 1.25 mg / day), which is treated with hormone impan (50 mg estradiol and 100 mg of testosterone) for 3 months. Libido improvement occurred in 80% of women, with reports of sexual response is better or equal to the time before menopause.[2]

Cardozo et al. (Al-Azzawi, et.al 2009) describe the effects of hormone implants subcutaneously in pre and postmeopause 120 women who came to the clinic menopause. A total of 67 postmenopausal women receiving 286 implants (50 mg estradiol and testosterone 100 mg every 4-12 months) for 4 years. The cure loss of libido reported on 67 women who lost their libido just before the start of treatment. In another study, Dow and colleagues, evaluated the testosterone implants (100 mg) with estradiol implant therapy (50 mg) compared with single estradiol implants in postmenopausal women who experience a decrease in sexual interest. There is no significant difference between the two group. [2]

Burger et al. (Sood R, et al, 2011) compared the efficacy of a combination of 100 mg testosterone implants and 40 mg of estradiol compared with a single 40 mg estradiol in postmenopausal women (either spontaneously or due to surgery) that has decreased libido during the use of progesterone and estrogen. At 6 weeks, improved libido and sexual pleasure recorded in women who treated with testosterone, and the improvement lasted until 18 weeks.[32,34]

In Indonesia, the management of testosteron insuficiency in menopausal women can be seen in this chart below, where they divide into first level of management, and if it failed, it has to be referred to second level of management which is usually performed by a gynaecologist.

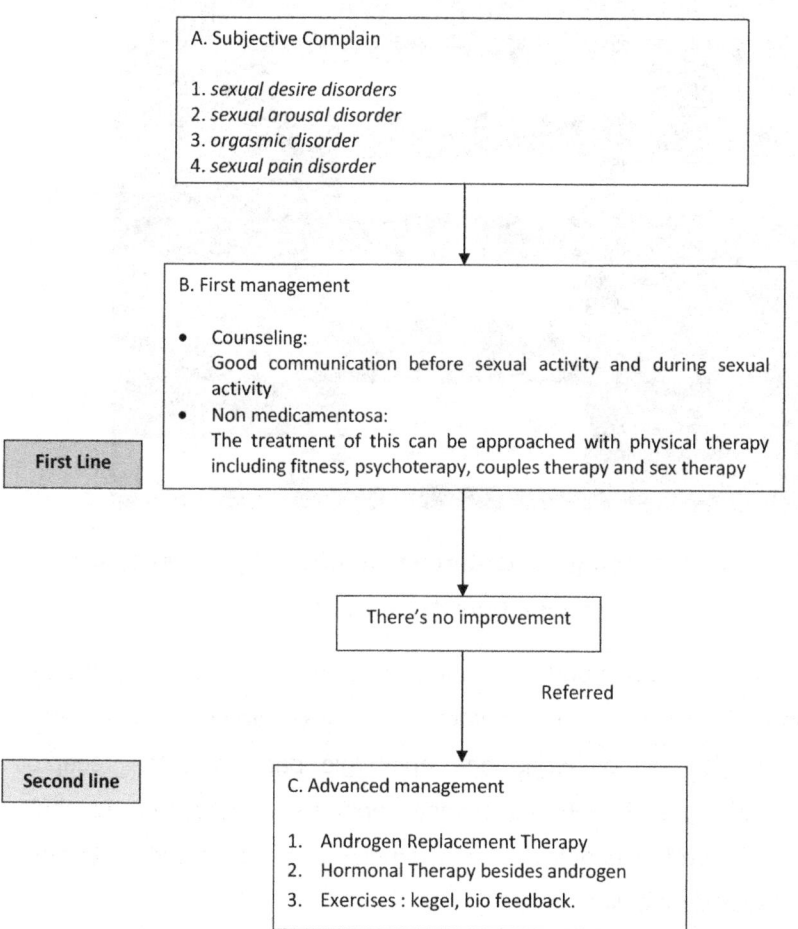

Figure 11. Chart Of Management For Testosteron Insuficiency In Menopausal Women In Indonesia[21]

While Bachmann et al made an algorithm to ease us in managing sexual dysfunction caused of testosterone insuficiency, as seen in figure below[35]

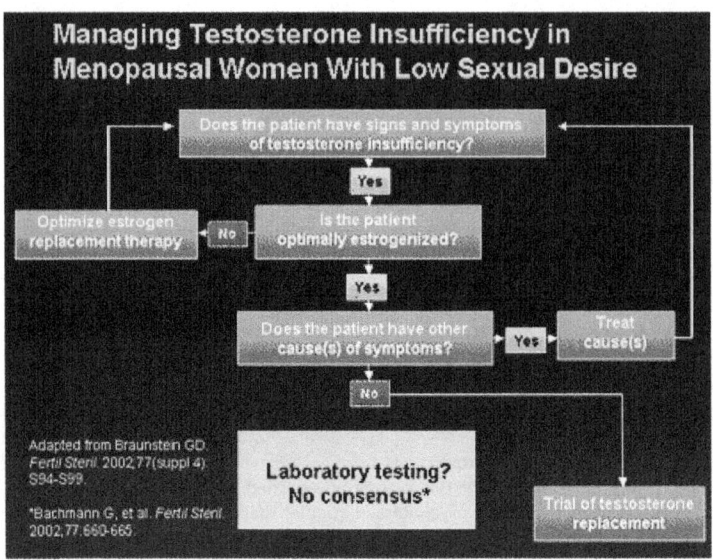

Figure 12. Managing Testosterone Insufficiency in Menopausal Women with Low Sexual Desire[35]

Androgens play an important role in sexual desire, arousal, orgasm and satisfaction by interacting with receptors in the hypothalamus, together with the dopaminergic, serotoninergic and opiatergic path, and the receptor genitals. Combining androgen and estrogen appears to increase a woman's sexual function, evidence obtained from studies in patients with estrogen-only, when testosterone was added.[5]

Sherwin et al. (Graziottin A, Serafini A. 2011) showed that women who received the combination therapy of estrogen / testosterone experienced a greater increase in sexual arousal compared with those who received estrogen only. Sarrel et al. indicate that estrogen only is not enough to resolve with all aspects of sexual function. Methyltestosterone adding estrogen to produce a significant improvement in sensation, desire and frequency of sexual activity. Somboonporn et.al. is reviewing the available literature on this subject and assess trials involving 1,957 patients. Estimates collected from the study showed that the addition of testosterone to hormone treatment (HT) improves sexual function score for menopausal women. The author of this review concluded that there are benefits of combining androgen to estrogen in terms of sexual function. However, the study looks at the meta-analysis using different testosterone regimens, making it difficult to estimate the effect of testosterone on sexual function in association with HT.[5]

A randomized, double-blind and controlled by Kocoskda showed no significant effect of testosterone or estrogen treatment for four weeks on verbal memory, verbal fluency, or spatial abilities in healthy natural postmenopausal women. HT, so that similar serum levels of sex hormones such as in this study, suggesting important clinical effects. Estrogen is the most effective treatment for the relief of menopausal symptoms such as flushing, sweating, and sleep disorders. Estrogen is also used for osteoporosis prevention and treatment of vaginal dryness and dyspareunia. Testosterone therapy has been proven improving psychosexual functioning and well-being in postmenopausal women who experience sexual desire disorder. However, they failed to find support sex hormones affect cognitive performance. In a study in women with hypopituitarism-androgen deficiency, they did not find the effect of testosterone in the treatment of cognitive function.[21]

A number of studies also have examined the effects of testosterone treatment on psychological variables in surgery or natural postmenopausal women. Several studies have assessed the effectiveness of testosterone treatment by using parameters such as mood, well-being, vitality. Improvement of these parameters have been reported in several studies after the use of testosterone.[5]

Results of a randomized controlled trial study concluded that testosterone therapy has the additional advantage for postmenopouse women when compared with the use of a single hormone therapy.

Advantages of changes including effects on sexual function, mood, bone density and increased body mass. Based on clinical data, the potential risk of side effects of testosterone, including acne, facial and body hair growth, deep voice, increased weight, emotional changes, and adverse effects on lipid profile. Lower high-density lipoprotein cholesterol (HDL), increased hematocrit, and abnormal liver function tests reported increased at higher dose oral methyltestosterone. The incidence of toxic hepatitis in a study including 572 794 women who were exposed derivative of oral estrogen plus methyltestosterone is 3 per 100,000 people per year. Long-term effects of testosterone on breast and other cancers, cardiovascular disease, and stroke is unknown. Because androgens converted into estrogen in vivo, potentially adverse effects of estrogen also affects the androgen therapy, such as effects on the breast and endometrium[24].

CHAPTER 4

CONCLUSION

According to WHO, menopause is the cessation of the menstruation cycle forever for women who had period monthly before, caused by the increasing numbers of follicles undergoing atresia until there is no more follicle left, and for the last 12 months do experience amenorrhoea that was not caused by pathological causes. Nowadays, Indonesian women experience menopause at approximately age 50. Nevertheless, some experience it in the early or late age. Age timing of menopause is influenced by heredity, general health status, an life style.

Examination of physical factors, psychological, cultural, and sexual relations affect the well-being and sexual function. Therefore, women who experience a decrease in sexual interest with or without interruption of sexual response should be assessed for psychological health, physical, and social in general. Stress , fatigue, relationship problems, depression, and common side effects of treatment contribute to a reduced sexual interest. When a woman enters menopause, physical discomforts such as stiffnes and pain could occur suddenly in the whole body. This stiffness is sometimes accompanied by a feeling of heat or cold, dizziness, headcache, fatigue, restless, irritable, and palpitations. After menopause, women will experience senile period. At this time, they reach a new hormonal balance so that there is no more vegetative or psychological disorders.

The use of testosterone in women is most often considered in postmenopausal women, while women have symptoms such as reduced sense of comfort, low libido, unexplained fatigue, decreased muscle strength, and changes in cognition or memory, all sof this called "female androgen insufficiency".

Results of a randomized controlled trial study concluded that testosterone therapy has the additional advantage for postmenopouse women when compared with the use of a single hormone therapy. Advantages of changes including effects on sexual function, mood, bone density and increased body mass.

AUTHOR

Muhammad Fidel Ganis Siregar MD, Ph.D., was born in Medan, Indonesia, 30 May 1964. He completed his medical degree in 1988, Specialist in Obstetrics & Gynaecoloy in 1997, Master Degree in Medicine and Doctor in Medicine in 2012 from Faculty of Medicine, Universitas Sumatera Utara, Medan Indonesia. Certified as Consultant in Reproductive Immunoendocrinology and Fertility Medicine from Indonesian College of Education in Reproductive Immunoendocrinology and Fertility Medicine. He is a lecturer in Graduate Programs in Faculty of Medicine, also for obstetrics & gynaecology specialists programs - Master of medical science programs and Doctoral in Medicine programs in the Faculty of Medicine, Faculty of Nursing, and School of Public Health in Universitas Sumatera Utara, Medan, Indonesia. As an Obstetrician & Gynaecologist many research has been done in the field of reproductive health, particularly those related to women's health and menopausal women. He won the title as the best Lecturer in Faculty of Medicine and also in Universitas Sumatera Utara in 2013. Also, he got a Travel Grant Award from the Asia Pacific Menopause Federation at a scientific meeting in Tokyo in 2013. In 2014, he receives Satya Lencana Karya Satya 20 Tahun, for 20 or more years of service to Indonesian government by President of Republic of Indonesia Susilo Bambang Yudhoyono. Currently he is the chairman of the Indonesia Menopause Society (PERMI) for Medan Region, a member of the division areas of the community service in Fertility and Reproductive Endocrinology Society of Indonesia (HIFERI), a member of Indonesian Society of Obstetrics & Gynaecology (POGI) and also a member of the Indonesian Doctors Association (IDI) until now.

REFERENCES

1. BlueCross BlueShield of North Carolina.. Hormon Pellet Implantation For Hormon Replacement Therapy in Women.2014. available from URL: https://www.bcbsnc.com/assets/services/public/pdfs/medicalpolicy/hormone_pellet_implantation_for_hormone_replacement_therapy_in_women.pdf
2. Al-Azzawi, et.al. Therapeutic options for postmenopausal female sexual dysfunction. In: Climaceteric. International Menopause Society. 2009.p 1-18
3. Australian Menopouse Society. Menopouse-Combined Hormon Replacement Therapy. Australasian Menopause Society Limited.2014.available from URL : https://www.menopause.org.au/for-women/information-sheets/23-menopause-combined-hormone-replacement-therapy
4. Velarde, Michael C. Mitochondrial And Sex Steroid Hormon Crosstalk During Aging. In: Biomed Central. 2014. Available from URL: http://www.ncbi.nlm.nih.gov/pmc/articles/PMC3922316/
5. Graziottin A, Serafini A. Medical Treatment For Sexual Problems In Women. Mulhall J.P .(Ed.) Incrocci L. Goldstein I. Rosen R. (Ass. Eds), Cancer and Sexual Health, Humana Press, 2011, p. 627-641
6. Yasui T et al. Androgen in Post Menopausal Women. Departement of Reproductive Technology. Department of Obstetric and Gynaecology. The University of Tokushima Graduate School. Tokushima Japan. The Journal of Medical Investigation. Vol 59 2012
7. Anggraini R, Siregar MFG, Adenin I. Kadar Glutathion Peroksidase (Gpx) Sebagai Penanda Derajat Keparahan Keluhan Menopause Pada Paramedis Wanita Menopause Di RSUP. H. Adam Malik Dan RS.

Jejaring Medan. Universitas Sumatera Utara. Departemen Obstetri dan Ginekologi Fakultas Kedokteran Universitas Sumatera Utara Medan, Indonesia, Februari, 2014

8. Ramadha D. Karakteristik Wanita Menopause Pada Wanita Perokok Di Kecamatan Tanjung Balai Utara Kota Tanjung Balai. Universitas Sumatera Utara. 2009.

9. Tambunan E. Gambaran Pengetahuan Dan Sikap Wanita Usia 40-50 Tahun Tentang Menopause Di Wilayah Kerja Puskesmas Sigumpar Kabupaten Toba Samosir Tahun 2010. Universitas Sumatera Utara.2010.

10. Morawati S. Kadar β-Cross-Links Telopeptide pada Wanita Postmenopause dengan Osteoporosis atau Osteopeni. Departemen Patologi Klinik.Universitas Sumatera Utara. 2009

11. Harlow, Sioban D. Executive Summary of The Stages of Reproductive Aging Workshop + 10: addressing the unfinished agenda of staging reproductive aging. In: Menopause: The Journal of The North American Menopause Society. 2012. Vol. 19. No. 4.p 1-9

12. Fauci AS, Kasper DL, Braunwald E, Hauser SL, Longo DL, Jameson JL, Loscalzo J : Harrison's Principles of Internal Medicine, 17th Edition : McGraw Hills, 2008

13. Hale, G.E. Hormonal changes and biomarkers in late reproductive age, menopausal transition and menopause in: Best Practice & Research Clinical Obstetrics and Gynaecology Vol. 23. 2009. p.7–23

14. Camelia V. Sindroma Pasca Menopause. Fakultas Kedokteran USU. 2010.

15. Speroff. L, Fritz. M.A. Female Infertility.Clinical Gynecologic Endocrinology & Infertility, Lippincott Williams and Wilkins. 8th Edition.2011.p.106-156

16. Monash University. Menopause. 2010. available from URL : http://med.monash.edu.au/sphpm/womenshealth/docs/about-menopause.pdf
17. Mwampagatwa I, et.al. Morpho-physiological features associared with menopouse: recent knowledge and areas for future work. In: Tanzania Journal of Health Research. Sky Journal of Medicine and Medical Sciences Vol. 2(8), 2014. pp. 058-066
18. Bentzen J.G., et.al. Maternal menopause as a predictor of anti-Mullerian hormon Level and antral follicle count in daughters during reproductive age. Oxford University Press on behalf of the European Society of Human Reproduction and Embryology. Vol.0, No.0 pp. 1–9, 2012
19. Reid, Robert. Managing Menopause. In: Journal Obstetry Gynaecology Cancer Vol.36. 2014. S1–S80
20. Chelnokova, Anna. Menopausal Symptoms and Complementary Health Practise in: National Institute of Health. National Cener for Complementary and Alternative Medicine.2013. Available from URL: http://nccam.nih.gov/health/menopause/menopausesymptoms
21. Perkumpulan Menopause Indonesia. Tatalaksana Gangguan Seksual. Konsensus Pencegahan dan Tatalaksana Menopause dan Osteoporosis. Jakarta. 2011
22. Speroff, L., Glass, R.H., Kase, N.G., Clinical Gynecologic Endocrinology and Infertility, 7th ed., Lippincott, Williams & Wilkins, 2004
23. Ambrose PJ. Drug use in Sports : A Veritable Area for Pharmacists. J Am Pharm Assoc. 2004;44(4)
24. Schwatz E, Holtorf K. Hormon Replacement Therapy in the Geriatric Patient: Current of the Evidence and Questions for the Future. Estrogen, Progesterone, Testosterone, and Thyroid Hormon

Augmentation in Geriatric Clinical Practice: Part 1. Clin Geriatri Med 27. 2011. p.541-559

25. Vermeulen A. Declining androgens with age: an overview. In: Oddens B, Vermeulen A, editors. Androgens and the aging male. New York: The Parthenon Publishing Group; 1996. pp. 3–14.

26. Somboonporn W, Bell RJ, and Davis SR. Testosterone For Peri And Postmenopausal Women (Review). In: The Cochrane Library. 2010.

27. Grohe C, Kahlert S, Lobbert K, Vetter H. Expression of oestrogen receptor alpha and beta in rat heart: role of local oestrogen synthesis. J Endocrinol. 1998 Feb;156(2):R1-7

28. Davis SR, McCloud P, Strauss BJ, Burger H. Testosterone enhances estradiol's effects on postmenopausal bone density and sexuality. Maturitas 1995;21(3):227–36.

29. Davis S, Davison S. Current perspectives on testosterone therapy for women in: American Society for Reproductive Medicine: Menopausal Vol 20. 2012.p.S1-S4.

30. Nappi R et al. Menopause and sexual desire . The role of testosteron. Menopause International. 2010.11: 16 : 162-168

31. Widjanarko B. Menopause. Available from URL: Reproduksiumj.blogspot.com/2009_11_01_archive.html.

32. Sood R, et.al. Counseling Postmenopausal Women about Bioidentical Hormons: Ten Discussion Points for Practicing Physicians. In: Journal Am Board Family Medicine Vol.24. 2011.p.202-210.

33. Monash University. Androgen in women. 2010. available from URL : http://med.monash.edu.au/sphpm/womenshealth/docs/androgens-in-women.pdf

34. Files J, Ko M, Pruthi S. Bioidentical Hormon Therapy. Mayo Clin Proc. Jul 2011; 86(7): 673–680.

35. Bachmann G, Bancroft J, Braunstein G, Burger H, Davis S, Dennerstein L, et al.Female androgen insufficiency: the Princeton consensus statement on definition, classification, and assessment. Fertility and Sterility 2002;77(4):660–5.

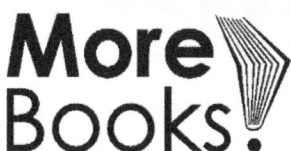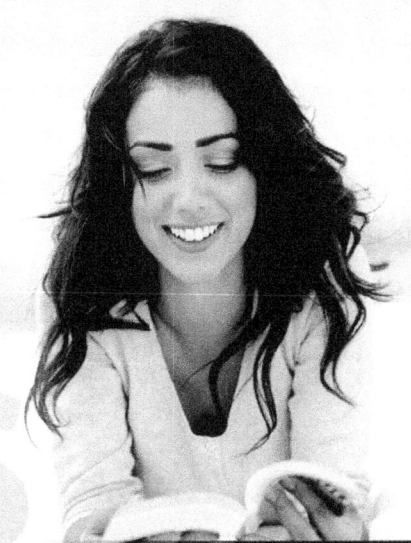

I want morebooks!

Buy your books fast and straightforward online - at one of the world's fastest growing online book stores! Environmentally sound due to Print-on-Demand technologies.

Buy your books online at
www.get-morebooks.com

Kaufen Sie Ihre Bücher schnell und unkompliziert online – auf einer der am schnellsten wachsenden Buchhandelsplattformen weltweit!
Dank Print-On-Demand umwelt- und ressourcenschonend produziert.

Bücher schneller online kaufen
www.morebooks.de

OmniScriptum Marketing DEU GmbH
Heinrich-Böcking-Str. 6-8
D - 66121 Saarbrücken
Telefax: +49 681 93 81 567-9

info@omniscriptum.com
www.omniscriptum.com

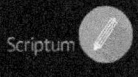

Made in the USA
Monee, IL
03 May 2026

49438545R00039